Laying Down the Armor: A Guide to Nervous System Regulation

By Miarah Jones, LCSW

Published by D Publishing Group™ Powered by D Investment Enterprise LLC

A Note Before You Begin

You are exhausted.

If you are reading this, you are likely the person everyone else relies on. You are the problem-solver, the rock, the one who holds it together when the world is heavy. You have survived 100% of your hardest days, and you have built a life through sheer force of will.
But survival is not the same thing as living. And the armor you had to wear to survive your past is now the very thing making you too heavy to move forward.

Trauma is not just a memory; it is a physical injury to your nervous system. It is the chronic tightness in your jaw, the sudden spike in your chest when the phone rings, the exhaustion that sleep doesn't fix, and the feeling that you are constantly waiting for the other shoe to drop.

You cannot out-think a nervous system injury. You have to feel your way out of it.

This workbook is not about being productive. It is not another task to add to your list. This is a somatic tool designed to bypass your overworked, exhausted mind and speak directly to your body. The intricate lines, the bilateral movements, and the grounding exercises here are scientifically structured to lower cortisol, engage your vagus nerve, and manually switch your brain from "survival mode" back to "safe mode."

How to Use This Space:

- **Put the armor down:** For the 15 minutes you spend on a page, you do not have to be strong for anyone.
- **There is no "Right" way:** Color outside the lines. Leave pages unfinished. Scribble over the words if you are angry. This book is a container for your healing; let it be messy.
- **Notice the shift:** Pay attention to your breath and your shoulders as your hands move across the paper. That quiet softening? That is the sound of your nervous system finally exhaling.

You have spent your whole life keeping everyone else safe. It is time to build a safe place for yourself.

In solidarity and healing,
Miarah Jones, LCSW

Published by D Publishing Group™ Powered by D Investment Enterprise LLC

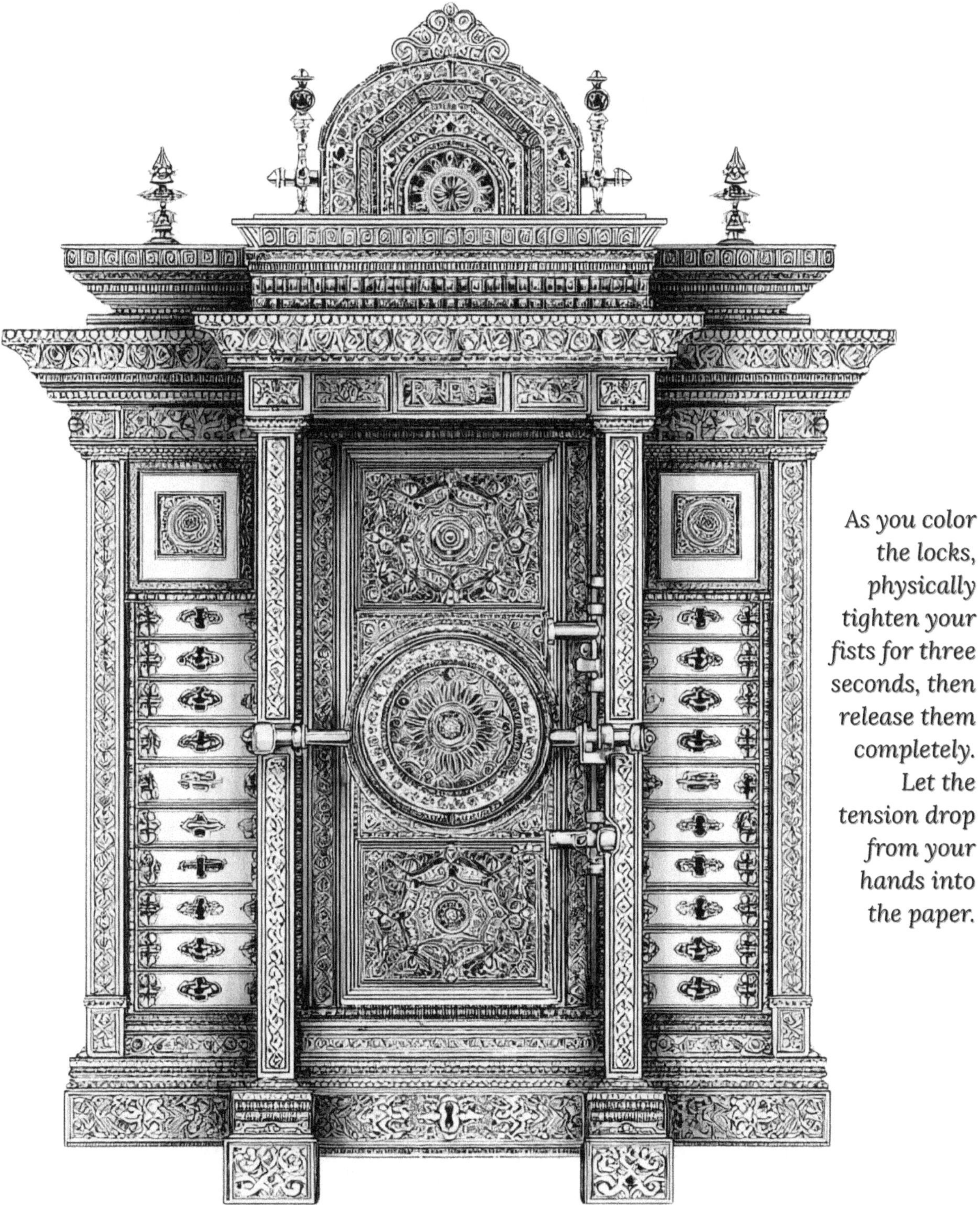

You do not have to process everything today. Sometimes, survival means putting the heavy things away so you can simply get through the afternoon. This is your container. It is infinitely strong.

Write the thoughts, memories, or stressors you cannot carry right now inside the drawers or the vault. Then, color the heavy locks. Leave it here. It will wait until you are ready and supported enough to open it.

Published by D Publishing Group™ Powered by D Investment Enterprise LLC

Reflections

Published by D Publishing Group™ Powered by D Investment Enterprise LLC

The Vagus Reset

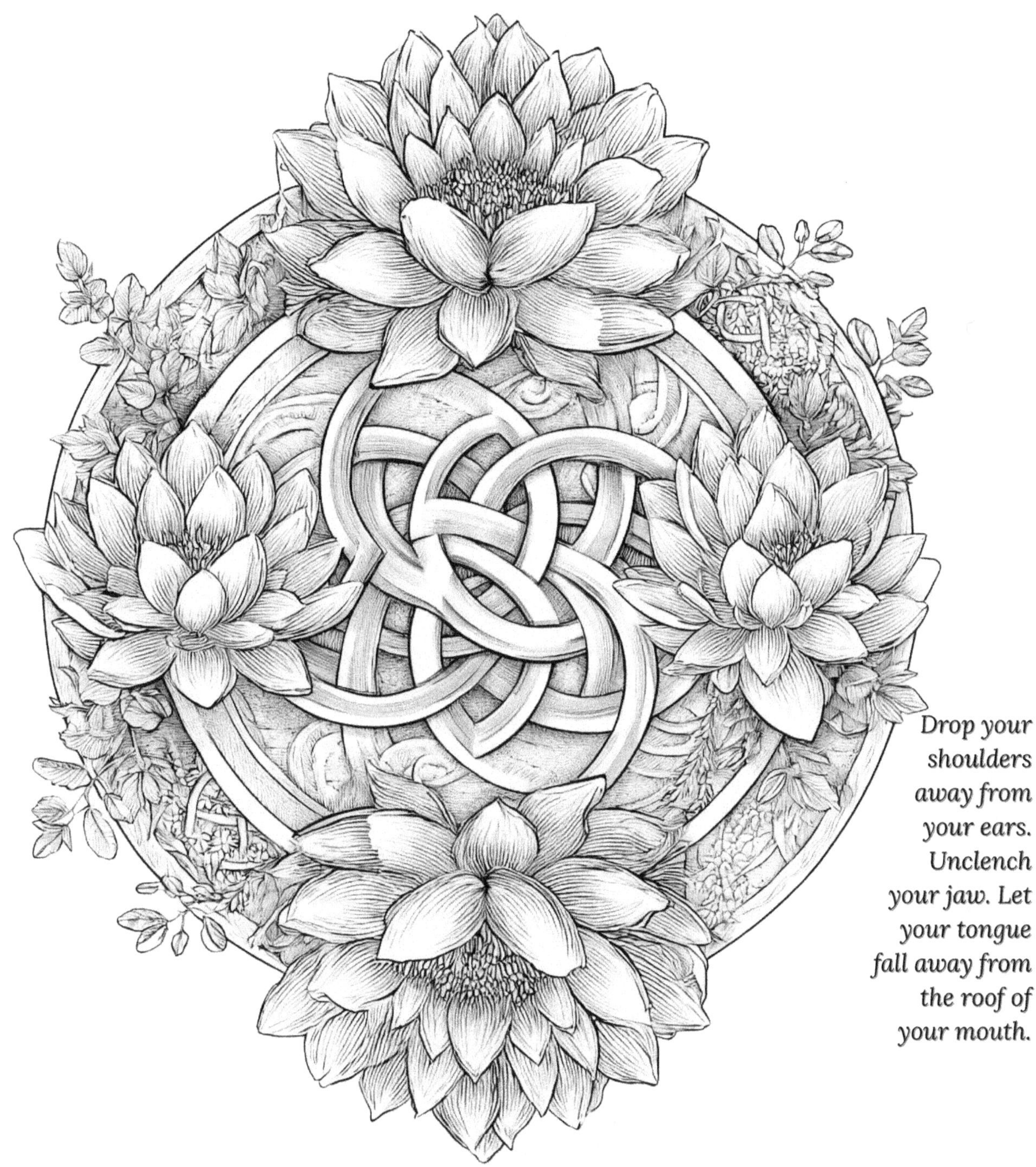

When trauma is triggered, your vagus nerve signals your body to prepare for war. We must manually signal that the war is over.

Trace the infinite lines of this botanical knot. As you color, purposely slow your exhale so it is twice as long as your inhale (Inhale for 4 seconds, Exhale for 8 seconds). The repetitive motion of your hand, paired with the extended breath, physically lowers your cortisol and heart rate.

Published by D Publishing Group™ Powered by D Investment Enterprise LLC

Reflections

The Protector

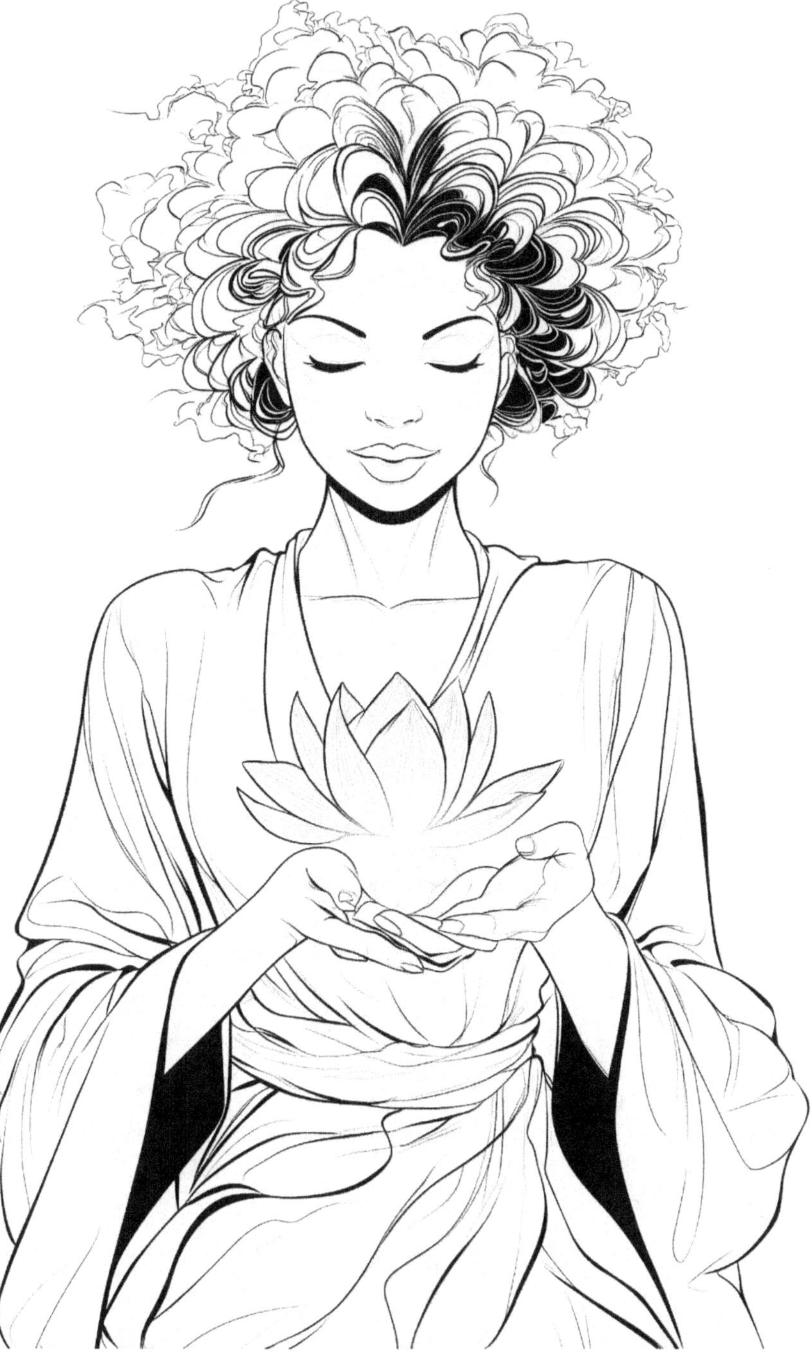

Place one hand over your heart and one hand over your stomach. Breathe softly into your hands while you focus on the image.

You survived by building armor. But the child who had to build that armor is still inside you, waiting to be told they are finally safe. You are the adult now. You are the protector they never had.

As you color this page, imagine sending warmth, safety, and permission to rest to the younger version of yourself. You do not have to fight anymore.

Reflections

Published by D Publishing Group™ Powered by D Investment Enterprise LLC

The Lineage of Resilience

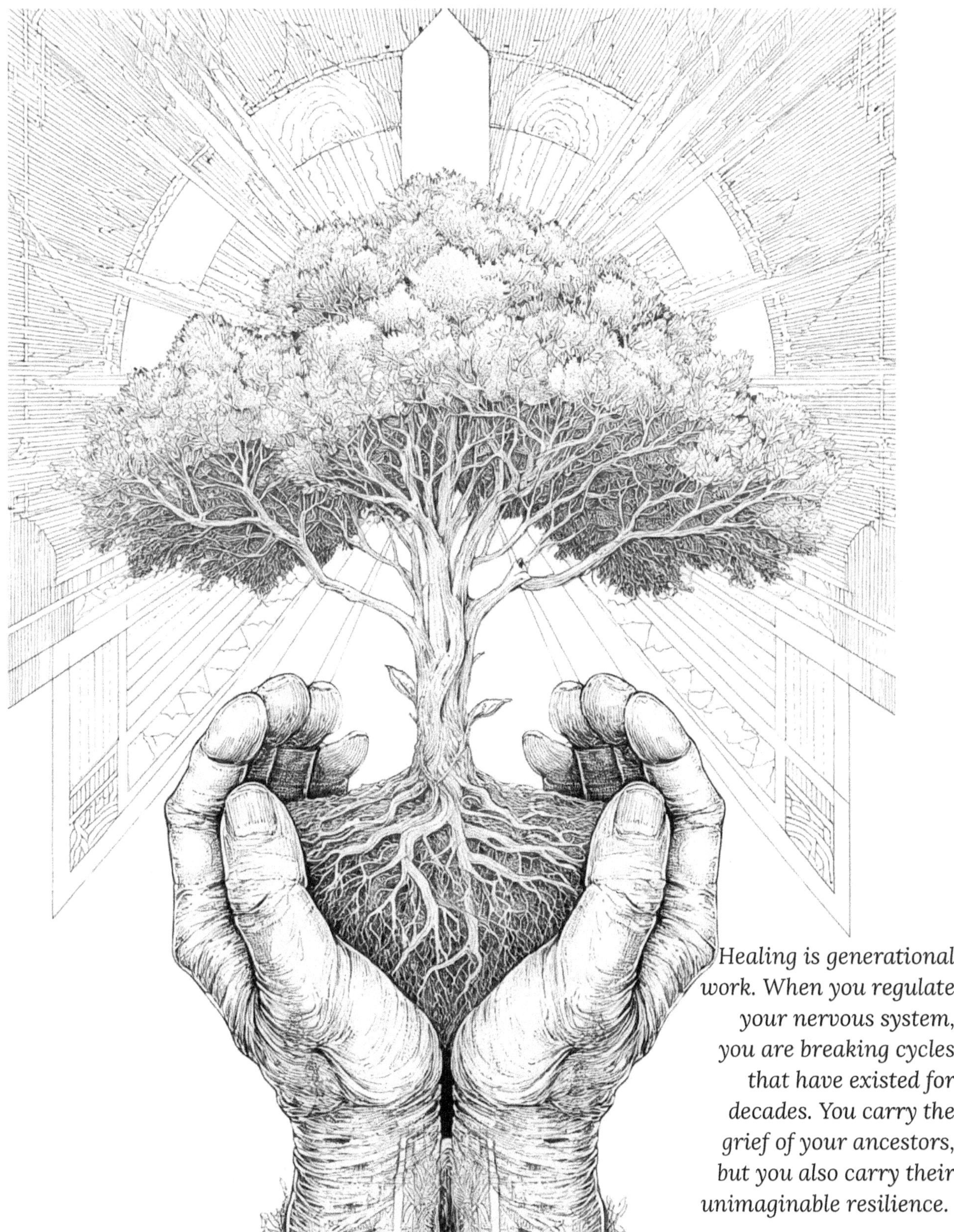

Write the names of those who came before you—or the strengths they passed down—in the roots. Shade the hands that planted the seeds, and color the canopy you are tending to today.

Published by D Publishing Group™ Powered by D Investment Enterprise LLC

Reflections

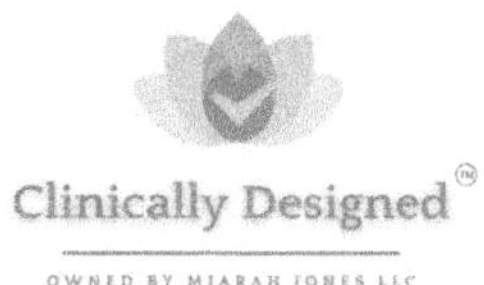

The Somatic Map

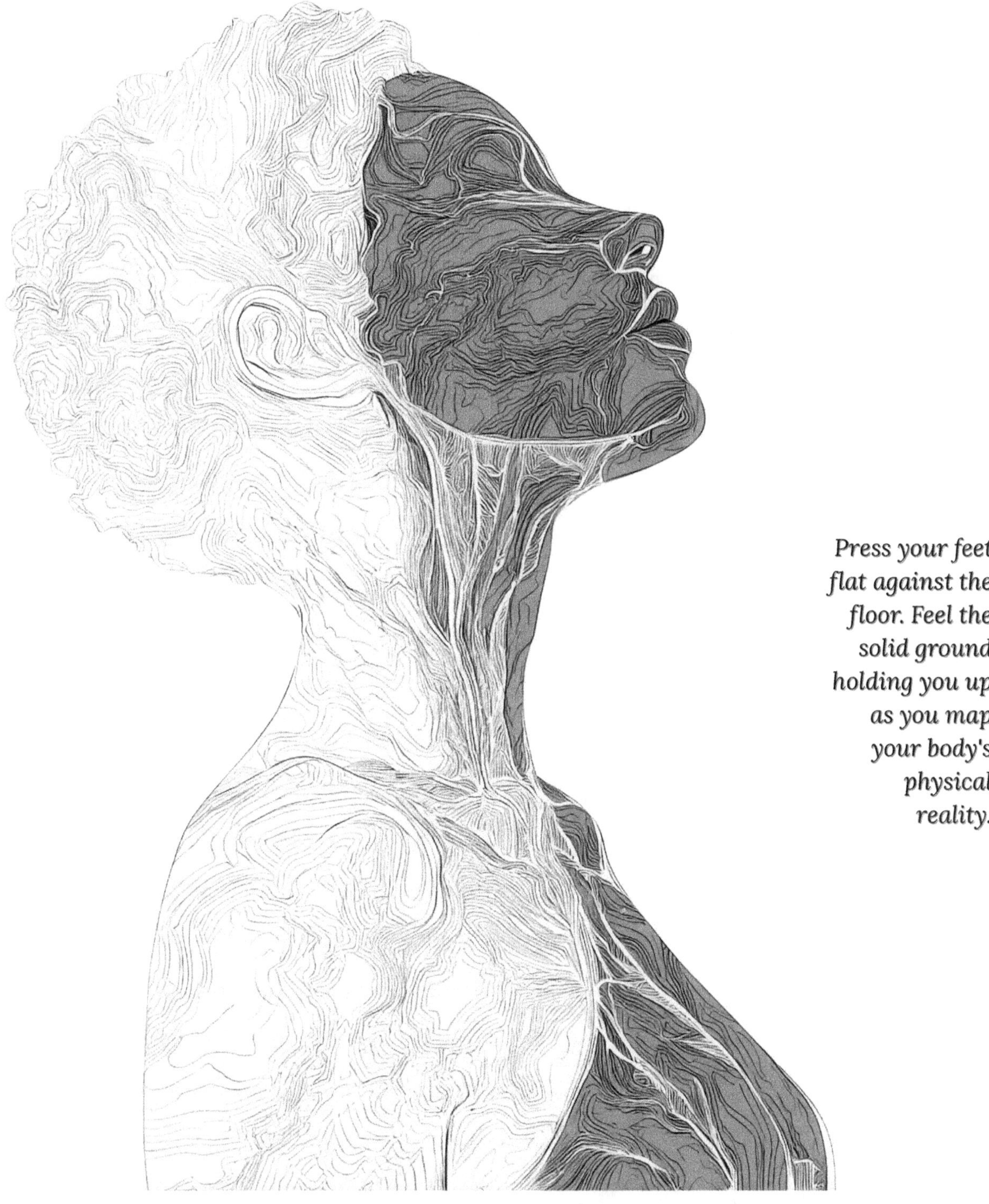

Trauma isn't just a memory; it's a physical weight. You cannot heal what you refuse to feel. Where are you holding the stress today?

Use dark, heavy colors to shade in the areas of this body where you feel tension, pain, or tightness (like your neck, chest, or hips). Use light, cool colors for areas that feel numb or disconnected. Map the energy.

Published by D Publishing Group™ Powered by D Investment Enterprise LLC

Reflections

Clinically Designed®
OWNED BY MIARAH JONES LLC

Published by D Publishing Group™ Powered by D Investment Enterprise LLC

The Pendulum

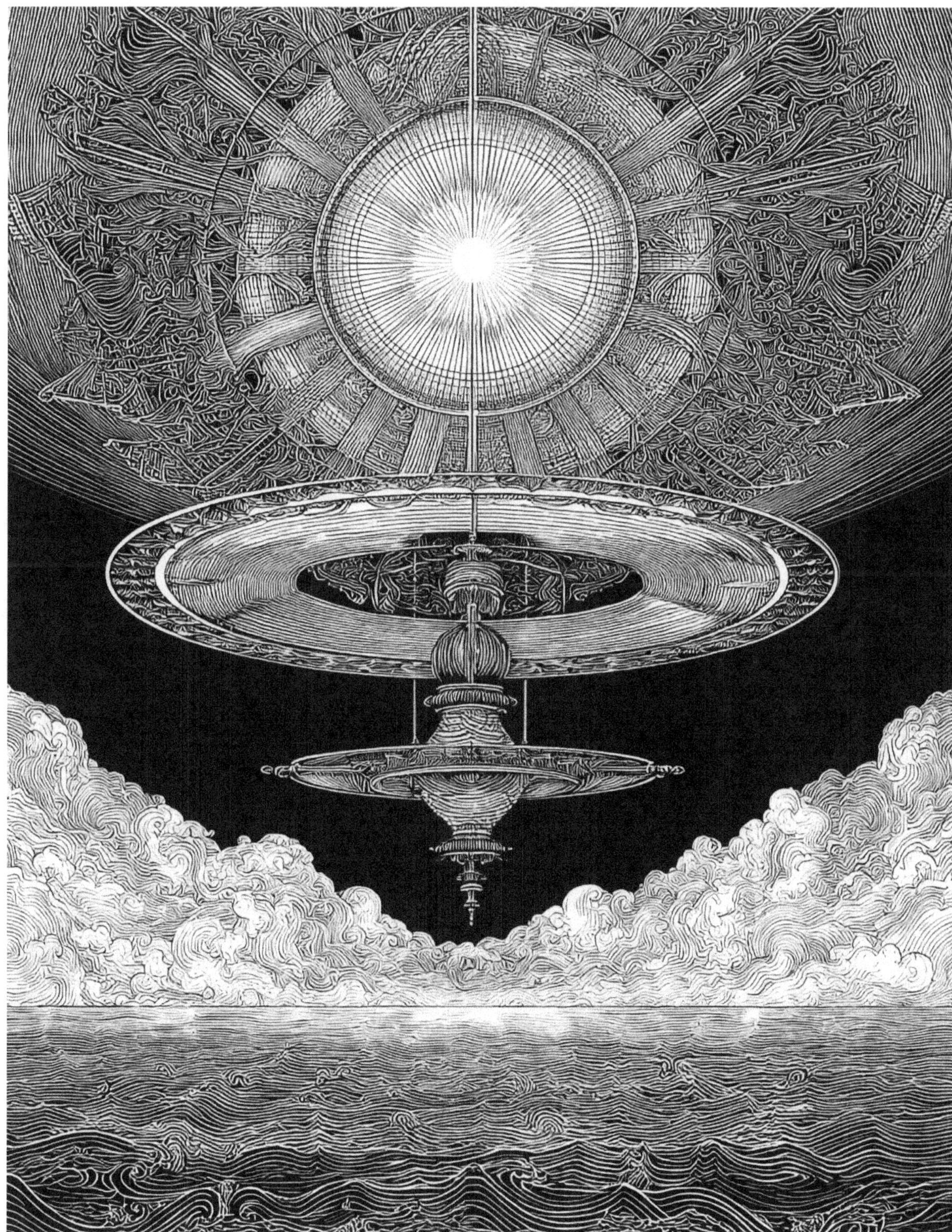

When your mind is racing, your brain's hemispheres are out of sync. Rhythm brings them back together.

Tap your left foot, then your right foot. Left, Right, Left, Right. Keep this steady, alternating rhythm going while you color the pendulum and the ripples. This bilateral movement crosses the midline of your body, helping your brain process and file away overwhelming emotions.

Published by D Publishing Group™ Powered by D Investment Enterprise LLC

Reflections

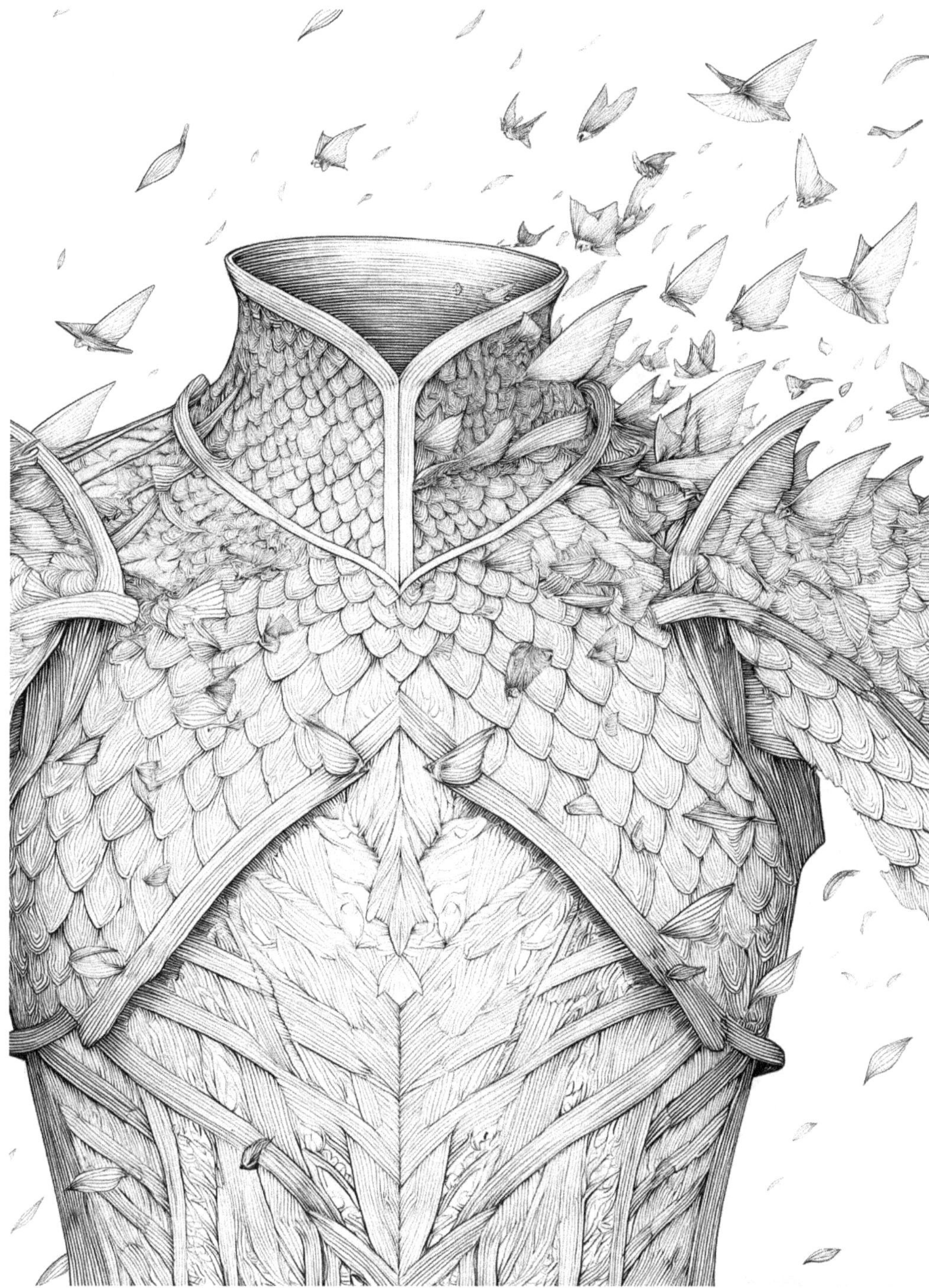

You have had to be the strong one for too long. Hyper-independence is a trauma response; it is the belief that no one will catch you if you fall. But right now, in this exact moment, you are safe. You do not need the armor here.

Color the pieces of the shield breaking away. Give yourself permission to put the heavy weight down, even if just for ten minutes.

Reflections

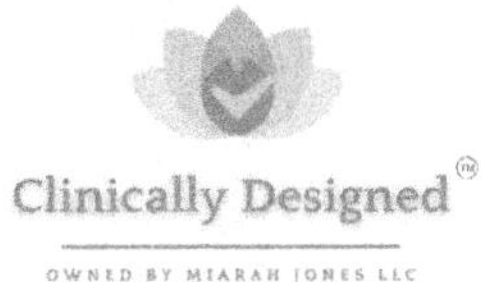

Published by D Publishing Group™ Powered by D Investment Enterprise LLC

The Anchor

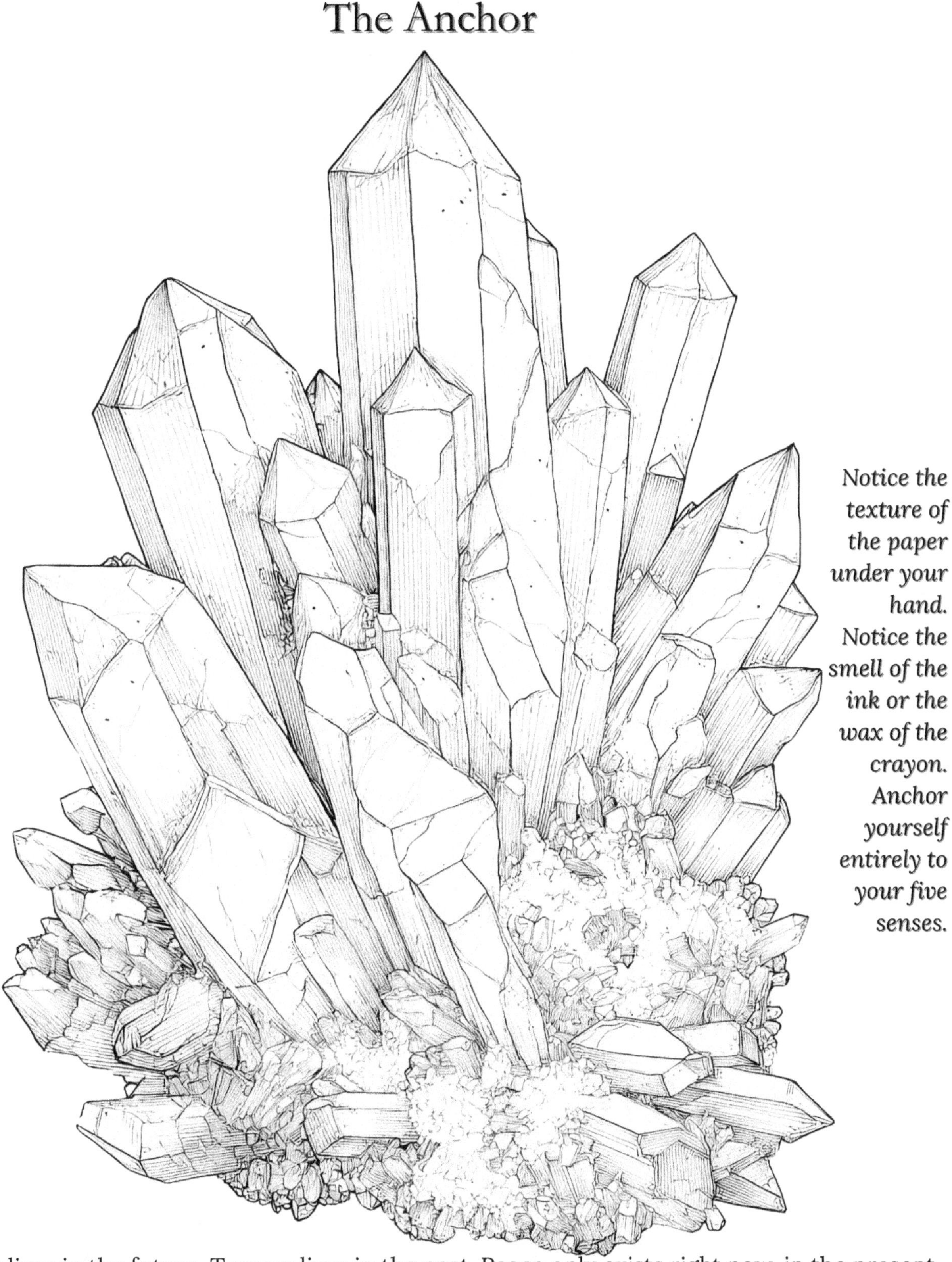

Anxiety lives in the future. Trauma lives in the past. Peace only exists right now, in the present moment. This geode has hundreds of tiny facets. To color it, you cannot think about tomorrow; you have to focus entirely on the space right in front of you.

Pick one tiny shape at a time. Color it completely. Stay right here.

Reflections

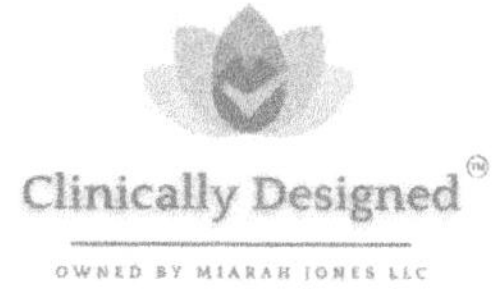

The Iron Gate

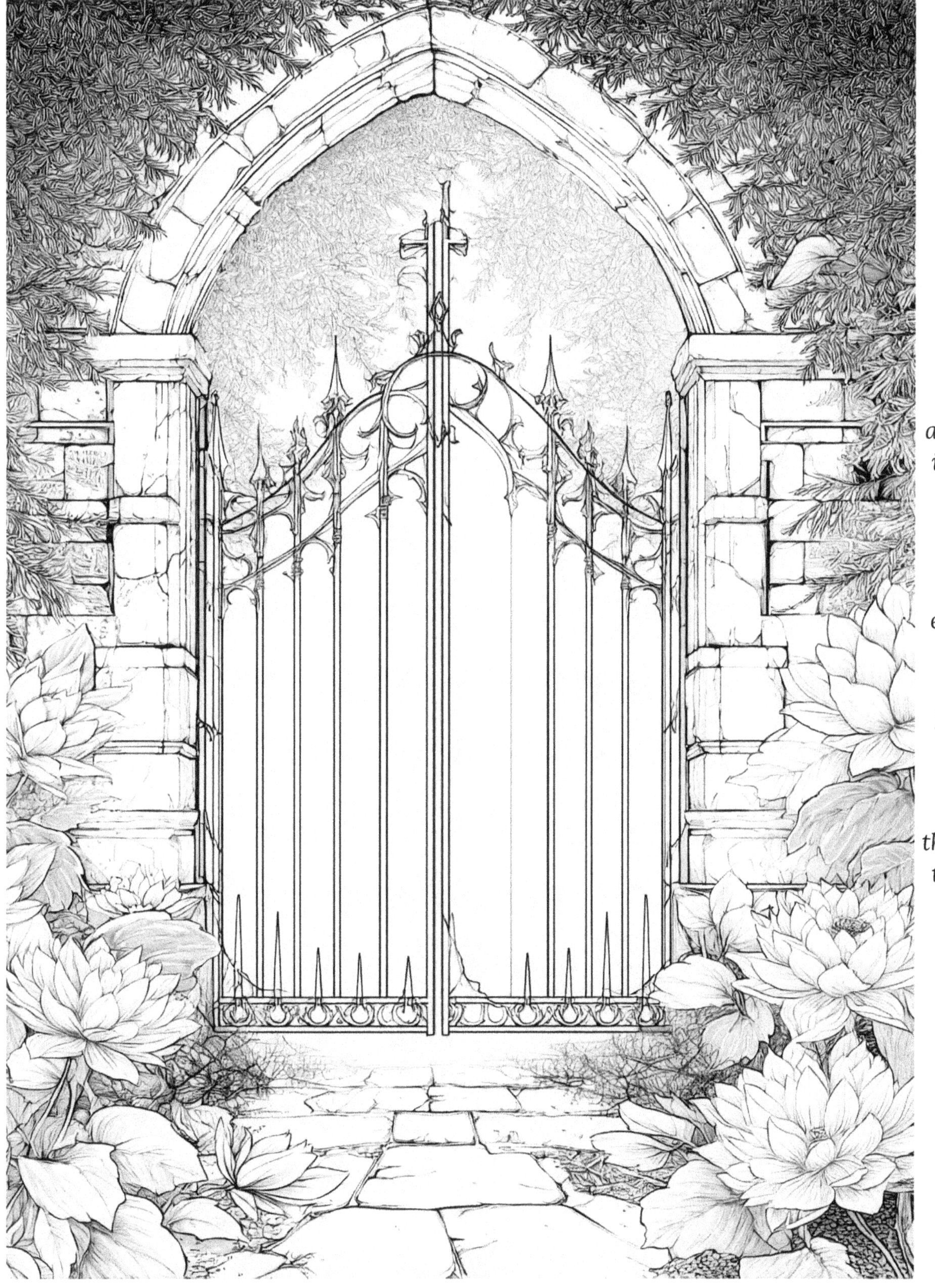

You are allowed to be inaccessible. You are allowed to say 'no' without an explanation. This gate represents your energy and your peace. Outside are the demands, the systemic pressures, and the people who drain you. Inside is your sanctuary.

Color the iron bars first, making them heavy, thick, and impenetrable. You decide who gets the key.

Published by D Publishing Group™ Powered by D Investment Enterprise LLC

Reflections

The Armor's Rest

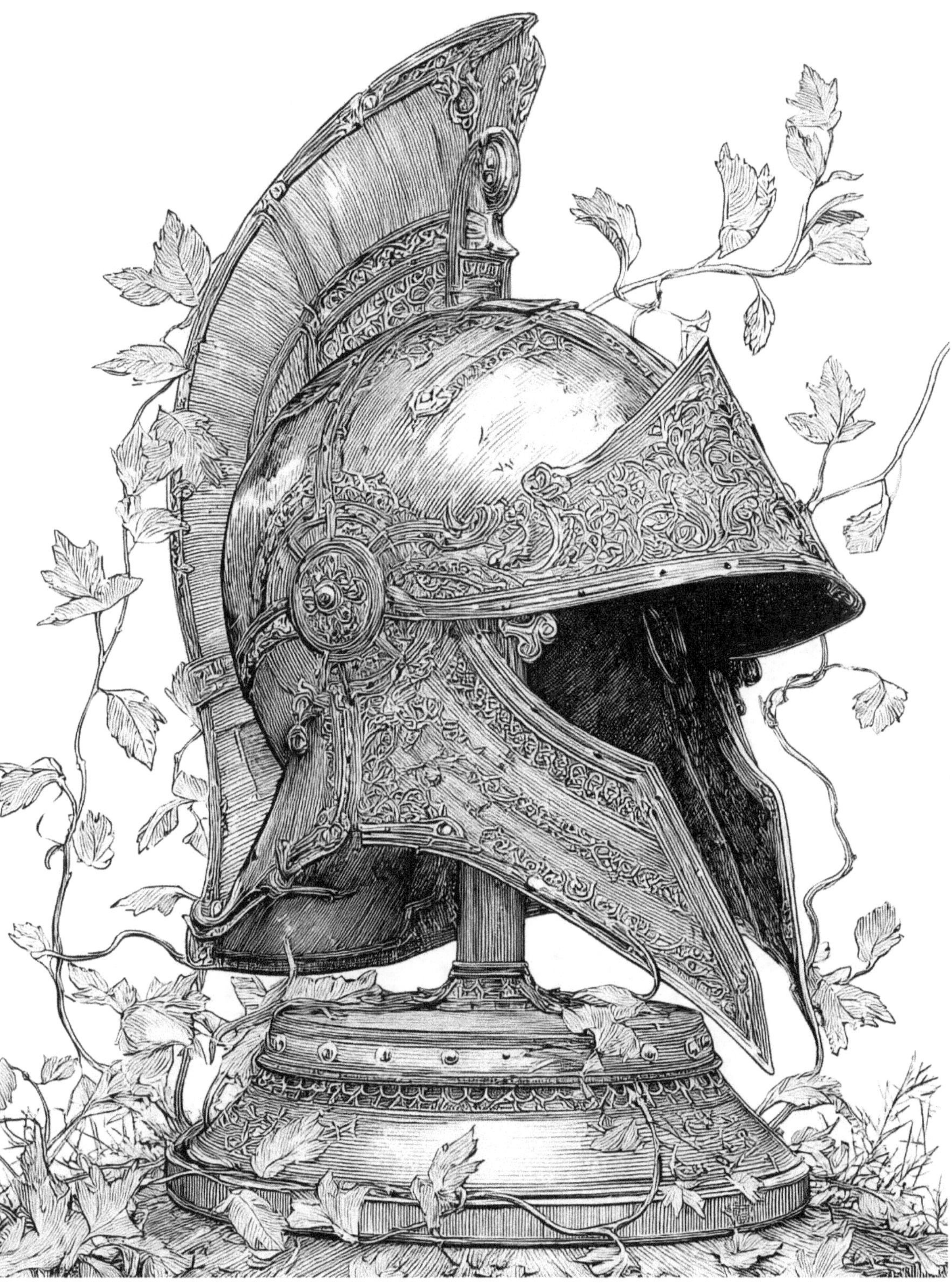

You have had to be the strong one for too long. You built this armor to survive a world that was not always kind or fair. It did its job, and it kept you alive. But it is incredibly heavy to wear every day. For the next ten minutes, you do not have to be strong. You do not have to protect anyone.

Color the armor, and give yourself permission to set it down.

Published by D Publishing Group™ Powered by D Investment Enterprise LLC

Reflections

The Mirror of Integration

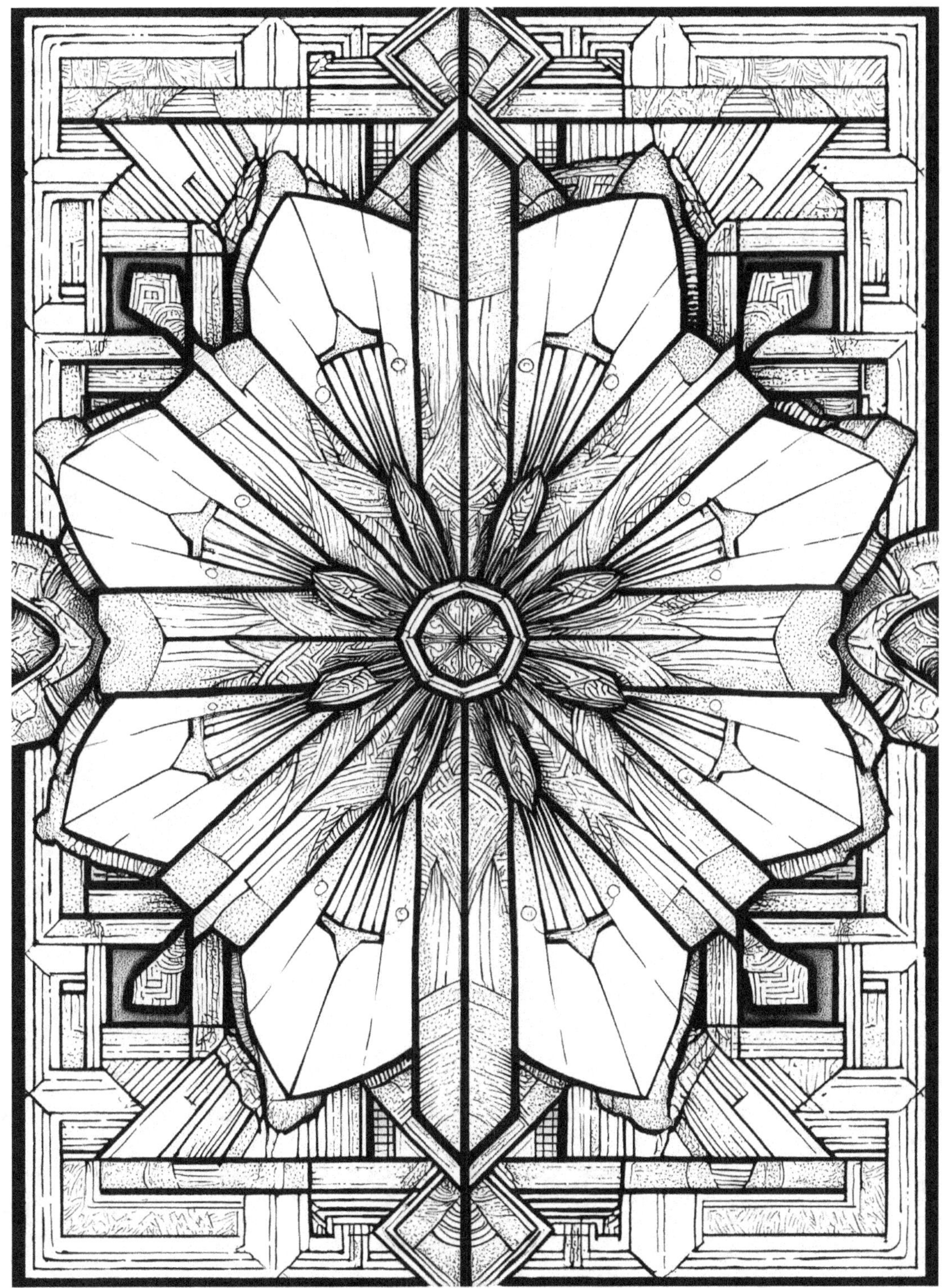

When a memory feels overwhelming, the right side of your brain (emotion) is overpowering the left side (logic). We need them to talk to each other.

Choose two colors. Keep one in your left hand and one in your right. Color one shape on the left side, then switch hands and color the exact same shape on the right side. Left. Right. Left. Right. Keep alternating until your breathing slows down.

Clinically Designed
OWNED BY MIARAH JONES LLC

The River's Carry

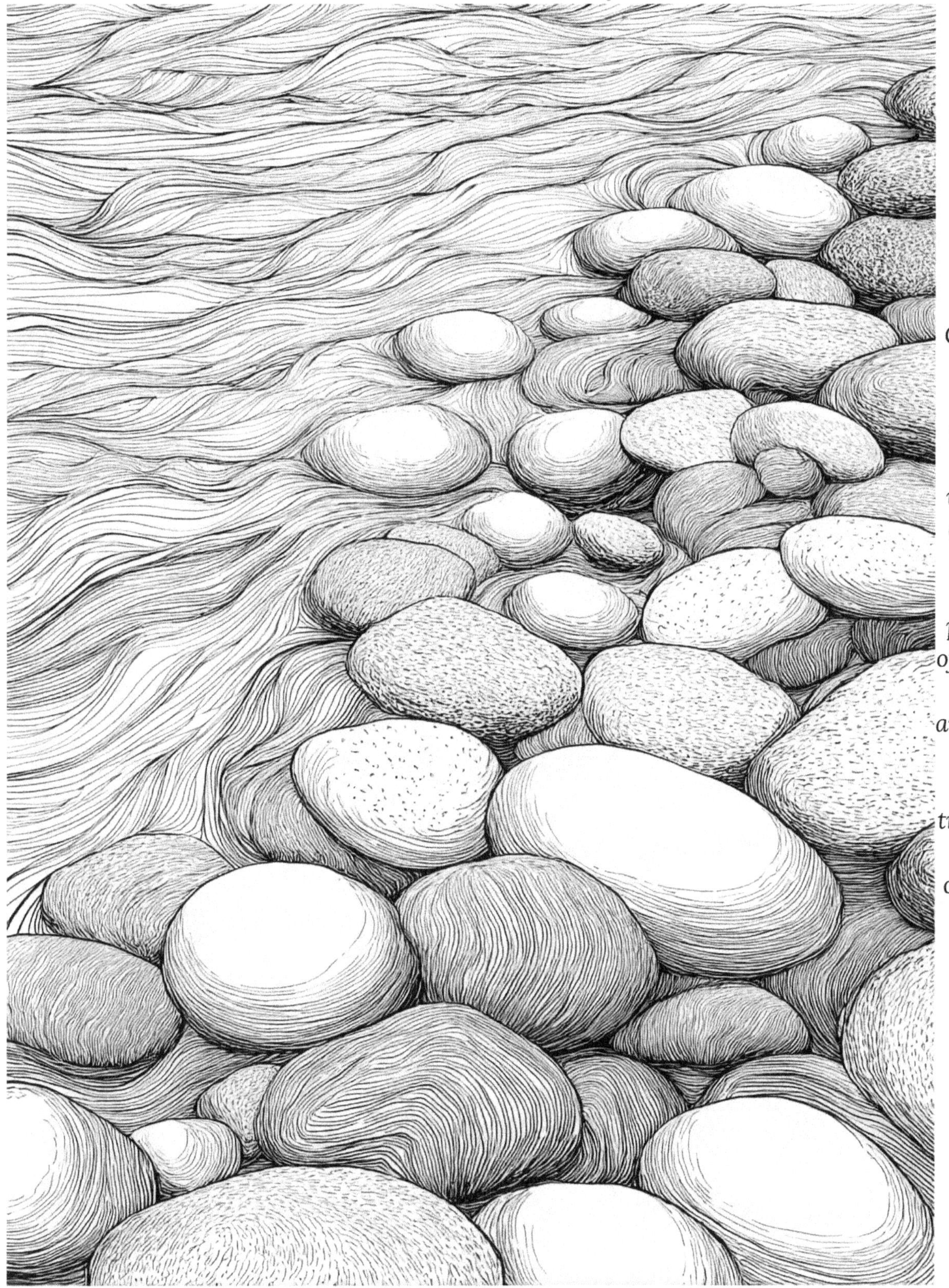

Grief is just love that has nowhere to go. When we swallow our grief, it turns into physical pain. Think of one heavy thing you are carrying right now. Imagine transferring the weight of that grief into these stones.

As you color the sweeping lines of the water, visualize the river washing over the stones, slowly eroding the pain and carrying it safely downstream. Let it go

Reflections

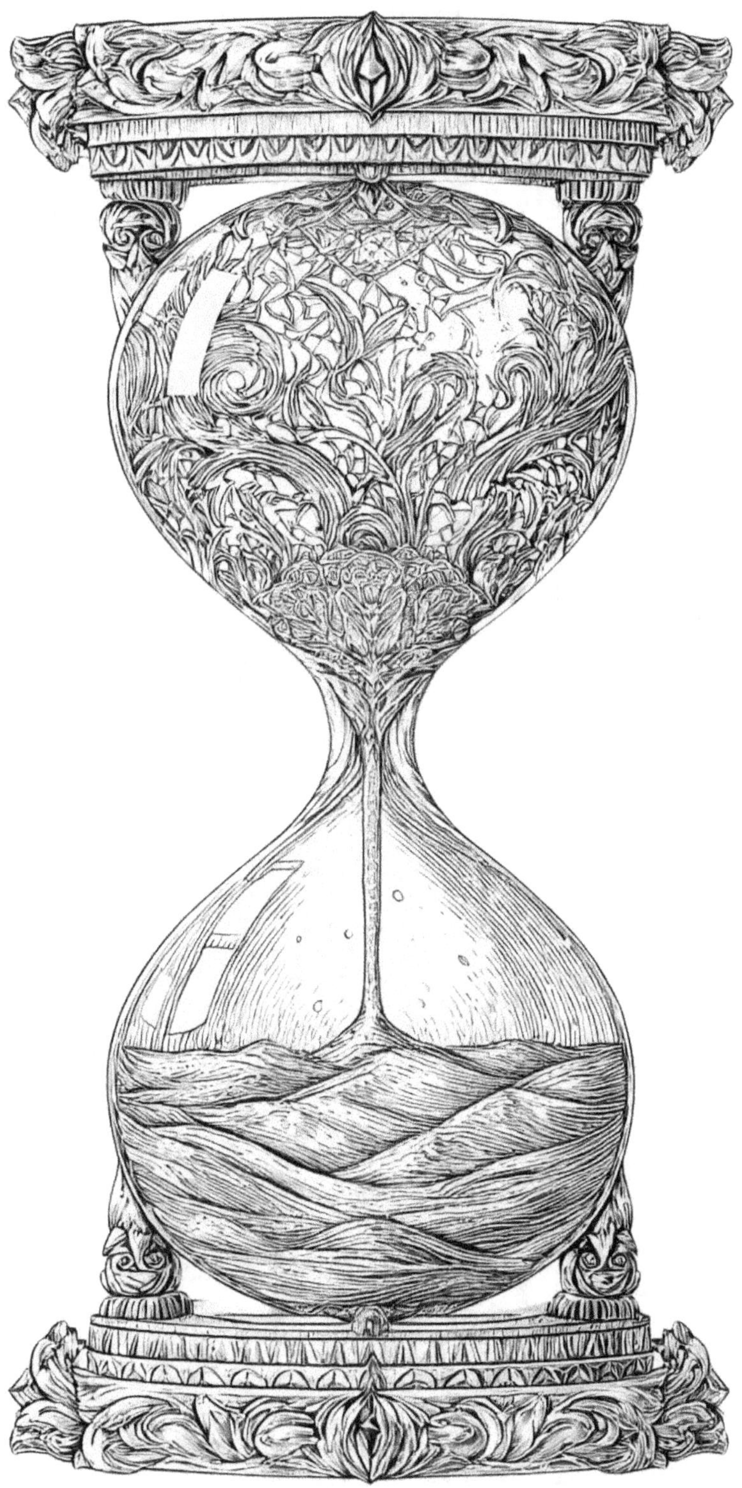

Trauma makes us react instantly because our brain thinks we are in danger. Healing is found in the pause. Between a trigger and your reaction, there is a split second where you have a choice. This hourglass is your pause.

As you color the chaotic lines at the top, take a deep breath in. As you color the smooth lines at the bottom, exhale slowly. Stretch the time out. You are safe.

Reflections

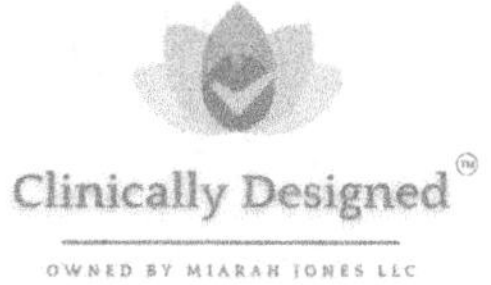

Clinically Designed ®

OWNED BY MIARAH JONES LLC

Published by D Publishing Group™ Powered by D Investment Enterprise LLC

The Steady River

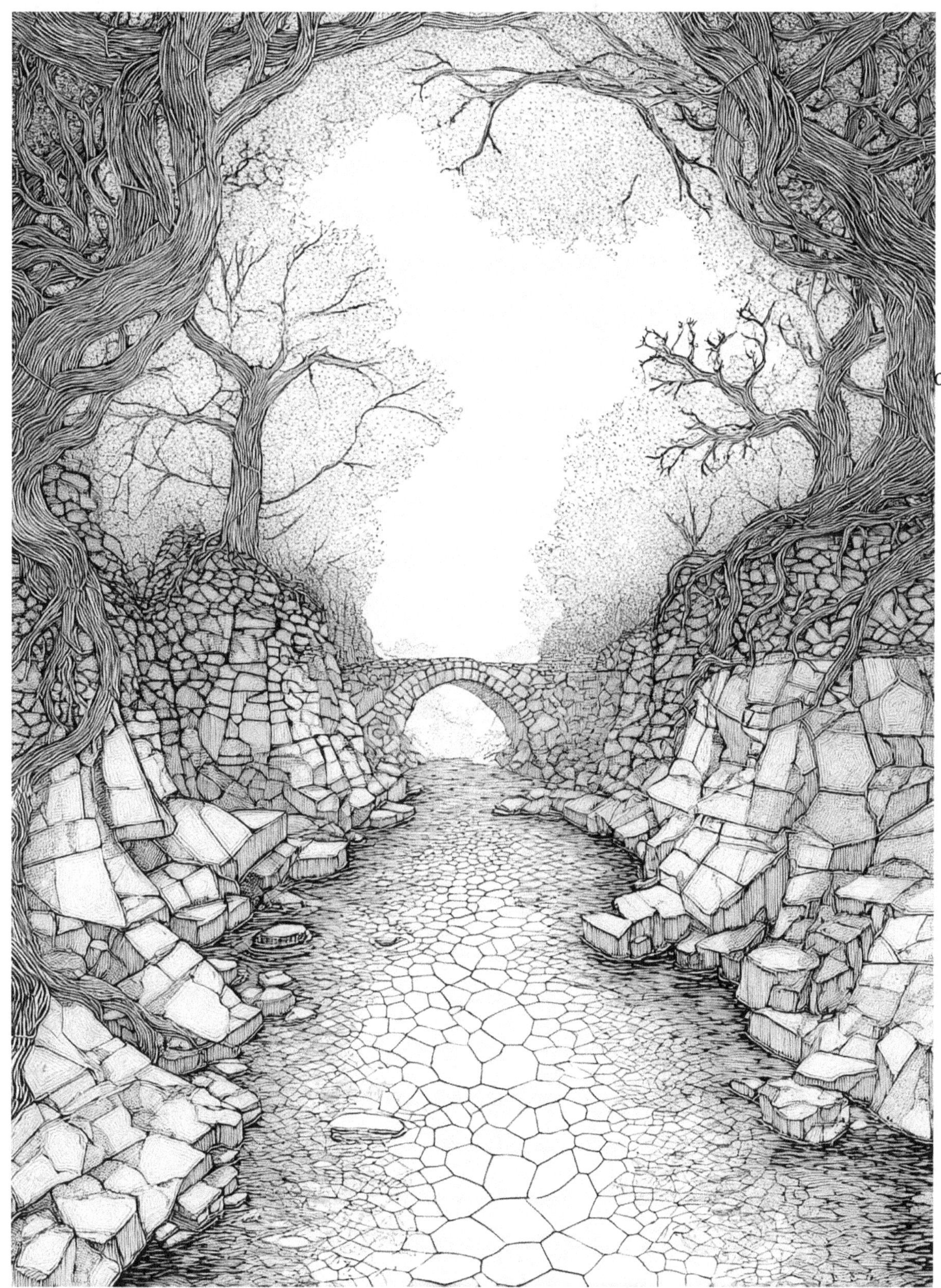

When your nervous system is overwhelmed, it either floods (anxiety, panic, rage) or freezes (numbness, exhaustion, shutting down). Healing is about widening your 'Window of Tolerance'— the space in the middle where the water flows smoothly.

As you color the river, focus on evening out your breath. You do not have to be a flood, and you do not have to be frozen. You can just flow.

Published by D Publishing Group™ Powered by D Investment Enterprise LLC

Reflections

Published by D Publishing Group™ Powered by D Investment Enterprise LLC

Published by D Publishing Group™

Powered by D Investment Enterprise LLC

ISBN: 979-8-9950444-4-4

Printed in the United States of America